<u>Why W.E.I.G.H.T?</u>

A six step weight loss system for frustrated female dieters

LEANNE HAWKER

DISCLAIMER INFORMATION

TABLE OF CONTENTS

PREFACE

Are there not a million books on weight loss already?

You're probably right, except there's probably a million and one. But the point is: there isn't a book like this book on weight loss! So, this is going to be different from the books that you've read before. Why? Because I'm sick of the BS we've been fed for years, and I am a woman on a mission and we all know that if a woman is on a mission it's pretty serious stuff!

Those million and one books probably treated you as just a number in a big pool of people looking to lose weight. This book is going to help you to find your individualised weight loss plan, which is really what you need, because one size just does not fit all, despite what slimming clubs will have you believe.

So why pick me? I've been in the fitness industry for about 20 years and my passion has always been about helping women to see that life does not have to be about endless cardio and limp lettuce and being on a permanent diet. Growing up I felt the pressure to look a certain way and that led me to a life of negative body image and very disordered eating. It certainly wasn't healthy and even when I was pregnant; I was told I wasn't eating enough, not on purpose, just as the result of a lifetime of diet marketing. It was having a daughter that made me decide to throw away the scales and show her that this was not the way. I even banned family members from talking about diets and 'fat days' around her. Have I succeeded – not entirely, those pesky diet fads and myths are very much still on her radar, it seems even I am not that powerful!

We're bombarded with weight loss everywhere we look. Women are scared to eat normally, feeling guilty because they eat a sandwich… (Fair enough, we all know that bread is an evil psychopath that will stick to your hips if you so much as pass it in the bakery aisle)! Not true by the way! It's confusing and expensive. There are far too many fads and quick fixes that leave you feeling like a failure and feeling despondent. From fat burning pills to meal replacement shakes, slimming clubs that have you counting points and relate foods to things you might take to confession, what the hell is the answer?

Did you know that the average woman spends around £25,000 pounds on dieting products and services in her lifetime?

Now I don't want to make you feel, sick but imagine what you could have done with that £25,000 pounds if you weren't so obsessed with hitting a target on the scales?

The diet industry has got it sewn up! It's a billion-dollar industry that helps you reach your goal quickly but doesn't give you the tools to be able to manage once you're out of the diet bubble and back in the real world. The weight starts creeping back on and then as if by magic, the next shiny new diet is laid out in front of you! This one will definitely be the answer to your prayers… this is it you think, ever hopeful! And the cycle continues.

In fact, weight isn't often even the real issue. You can reach your ideal weight and still be unhappy with your body. When I was younger, I wasn't overweight, but was constantly trying to lose weight because I felt I wasn't good enough as I was. I felt I didn't match the ideals that were being thrown at me all the time. Constantly looking at myself in the mirror and hating how I looked. And despite other people probably thinking there was nothing wrong with me I just couldn't see that for myself. Looking back through a different lens I can see what a massive waste of energy that was, but when you're trapped in the cycle it's hard to get out. It's the same with dieting and constantly trying to reach some stupid target weight that someone has decided you should be striving for! (FYI target weights are often miserable to achieve and not sustainable)!

So, my point there is that just because you reach your ideal weight that does not mean that you're then going to be happy with yourself. And this is often the place where women find themselves. They've been on a diet expecting that the minute they reach their goal weight, everything in life is going to fall into place, well it doesn't!

In fact, these days the world is changing, and weight loss can be a dirty word. We currently have two camps; body positivity and the gym body look and influencers all over are queuing up to jump on one or other band wagon!

With the body positivity movement sweeping the globe, it can almost put an umbrella of shame over people who still want to lose weight. Don't get me wrong, body positivity is absolutely a great thing and something that I constantly promote within my classes and the work I do with women, especially with the fact that my body image was terrible for most of my life. I do think that body positivity is a good thing, but I also do have a few little problems with it.

Firstly, it makes you feel ashamed if you don't already love yourself as you are. And I can tell you now that is no mean feat to achieve – take it from someone who knows. It's not easy to love yourself because as women we're constantly told that we're not good enough. Even if we manage to reach one societal ideal in terms of how we look, the next time we look we're meant to be something else. One minute we're meant to be waiflike with no butt and no boobs. The next minute we're meant to be all butt and boobs!

Secondly, it adds another element of shame to the idea of weight loss, as if people who are trying to lose weight don't already feel bad enough, now they must feel bad for wanting to make a positive change! Some so-called body positive influencers always seem to have a reason why they're bloated, or their stomach isn't flat. Which to me signals you're not necessarily entirely comfortable with your body because if you are why the justification?

I think that highlights how difficult it is for the average woman to have a positive body image, if even those who promote it all the time still struggle. And no matter how body positive you are, we can't deny that obesity does play a part in our health outcomes and longevity of our life and sometimes to the fullness of life that we lead.

These days, there's also a shift towards more of a workout body, but not your average pop to the gym a couple of times a week gym body; the sort of body that can only be achieved by going to the gym 5 days a week and miserably munching broccoli and chicken for 12 weeks before being smothered in a very orange tan and parading about on stage in sequins! Now don't get me wrong, I have nothing against anyone who wants to do this, I admire their dedication and I am partial to a sequin myself, but for most women this is unattainable. Not because they couldn't do it if they wanted to, but because most women don't have the capacity or will to take on this level of commitment. Whether you do or you don't, you will no doubt be looking at images of these women a lot, so again the goalposts for women are changing – it's no longer enough to just lose weight you must now have abs like a cheese grater!

However, you do not have to fit society's ideals to be fit and healthy.

This book is about taking you down a different weight loss path. One that sees you as an individual, one that doesn't follow a one size fits all approach. One that weeds out the BS we've all been inhaling for years.

I will help you to learn to enjoy the journey rather than feeling miserable until you get to the desired result. And I'll teach you how you can keep the weight off once you've lost it. Women who follow my advice have had good results and more to the point they haven't felt miserable or restricted. It can feel uncomfortable to follow a process which is completely different to the ones you're used to following and to untangle the diet mind-set you are used to, which is often the biggest hurdle to overcome in terms of losing weight and keeping it off.

So how will my book help you? Well, firstly, most of us don't want to just lose weight. What we actually want is to lose weight and keep it off. None of us want to be on the diet treadmill our entire lives, I'm pretty sure you don't wake up with a yee-haa on a Monday morning at the prospect of your diet starting AGAIN! And quite frankly we've probably got way better things we could be doing than constantly bouncing from one diet to another.

This book will help you to take your focus away from the weight goal and focus on the process which will be the key to ensuring that you are able to lose weight and to keep it off and make it fit your lifestyle. As I said at the beginning, this really is going to be a plan that you can make individual to you. It's not going to be the same as Susan three doors down or Brenda at work; it's going to be what fits your lifestyle, your needs and your non negotiables and that's the difference.

The good news is despite the years you've spent thinking it's not going to happen, it **can** happen.

Weight loss really doesn't have to be that difficult, but it's been made difficult by an industry that wants to make money from you. It doesn't benefit them to have you succeed. Oops I guess that's any sponsorship deals out the window. But seriously, it's the truth. Slimming clubs bring about disordered eating, (a banana mashed is still a banana), and the humiliation of group weight shaming in the form of weekly weigh- in. And if your diet means you're going to go to weigh in and then basically buy the entire cake aisle afterwards – that is not a diet plan that works!! Then we have 'skinny' beverages that might make you have a nasty bowel accident on the bus, all in the name of a couple of pounds weight loss before your holiday where no one knows you anyway. And that's just a couple of examples.

The fact that there are so many different options out there for weight loss also leaves you confused. Not sure which one is going to be the right answer. And that's why quite often you don't stick to anything for a consistent length of time because you've just started something and then the next new shiny diet comes out and off you go on to the next thing that you're sure will give you the answer this time. (I get it – I have shiny object syndrome too).

The fact of the matter is that the only real answer is to find something that is going to work for YOU. And that's what this book is going to show you how to do.

Throughout this book, we will look at the reasons why you're struggling to lose weight. What's going on in your mind around your weight loss, what diet myths are you taking on that aren't serving you? Learn how your time can be better spent than worrying about whether you ate at 6.01pm yesterday.

After we've worked on the diet myths, and your personal mind-set, we'll look at the things that are important to you. For example, whether you want to have that weekly take away with your family or a packet of crisps with your lunch every day. FYI one of my non-negotiables is having 2 chocolate biscuits every day if I want to. I will talk about the power of this simple trick later in the book.

I'll help you to see the things that you can compromise on and the things that you're adamant that you want to keep. I'm not going to lie to you, there does have to be an element of compromise. I wish we could eat a whole Victoria sponge cake every day and still be the weight that we want to be, but unfortunately, it's unlikely to happen. But the good news is we can still include those things and achieve our goals – you actually can have your cake and eat it!!

Chapter One

So, I know we've touched on the current state of the weight loss industry and the body image philosophy that currently is in play. But I thought I'd go into a little bit more detail on the topic.

In some ways, not much has changed for women with regards to how we feel about our bodies and our weight and the messages that we're given on a day-to-day basis. We are set unrealistic standards of how we should look. We're expected to weigh the same as we did when we were in our 20s pre children, pre menopause, pre anything basically! We spend our lives being presented with images of women who look the way that we are told we are meant to. But we're not told the true story, that these women are often airbrushed and in today's extremely modern technological society, they are now edited in so many ways that I can probably guess that even the models wouldn't recognise themselves if they saw these images of themselves. This pressure has been around for women for a long time. I remember reading magazines as a teenager and constantly being told about how I should look; what I should be eating; what diet I should be following. There is literally no women's magazine in the world that I have seen, and I'm open to being corrected, that does not feature a diet of some sort.

Magazines these days will be bigging someone up for their curviness on page 5 and selling a diet on page 6, telling you how to make a cake on page 13 and then slagging off some celebrity for having cellulite on the centre spread. Women just can't win no matter what we do. And sometimes our bodies just aren't meant to be a certain way. We're all different and we're not all going to look the same regardless of which diet or exercise plan we follow.

Not only are we meant to be whatever society tells us we're meant to be, we're now also meant to be okay with how we actually are. Confused? I am. We're meant to change but not want to change because we're supposed to be okay with our bodies and how they are. We're also expected to be in the gym lifting heavy weights and getting our bikini bodies without any excuses. So just when we thought it couldn't get any more confusing, it gets more confusing. And now we're not sure whether we should love ourselves as we are or change ourselves to something else!

We're not sure whether to embrace the cake aisle or avoid the cake aisle! To eat carbs or to not eat carbs? Are we allowed fat? Is fat good for us or bad for us? Should we completely ban sugar? Who knows? I don't know. No one knows. Even the diet industry itself can't make its mind up which is why things are changing all the time. Touching on that topic, we have crazy diets out there and we always have. Back in the 80s we had things like the cabbage soup diet. In the 90s there was the Atkins diet, where we had to eat a very low carb diet, cutting out foods that are actually good for us. We have people who claim that we shouldn't eat fruit because it's bad for us. People that claim that we should cut out all sugars because it's bad for us and of course they've had amazing experiences through doing that and we should all follow their lead. We should exercise, but we shouldn't exercise. We should exercise extremely. But then we shouldn't over exercise. We don't want to exercise because some diets tell us that if we exercise we're going to get heavier and of course weight is the only measurement of success. It isn't.

Do we spend hours on the treadmill? Or do we do 20 minutes of HIIT (High Intensity Interval Training) and hope that it's going to provide the desired result? Should we do both? Are we meant to work out morning and evening? Just once a day? Every day? Twice a day? Do we do weekends or not? We're not sure. And this is why the diet industry is BS for many of us, we're so caught up going around in circles and trying to decide what we should do that we're actually not doing anything at all. And through this we're gaining more weight and in turn this could be affecting our health, could be affecting our confidence and could be affecting how we live our life.

The issue is we have so many options now that we're never picking one and sticking with it consistently, instead constantly flitting from thing to thing, thinking that the next shiny new diet is going to give us the answer that we've been hoping for. Slimming clubs convince people that they have the answer. Then when you leave and the weight creeps back on, they convince you that you need them again, despite the fact that if it worked, you probably wouldn't be going back for the 10th time this year and for the next 10 years.

Successful weight loss plans should be about fitting in with your lifestyle, with your needs, with the things that you can manage on a day to day basis. It's about making a change for life. There is no point making changes that you are unable to sustain for the rest of your life because you will lose weight but not keep it off. Slimming clubs are pretty much about losing weight – end of story. They're not about keeping it off because if you keep it off, they've lost a customer and they want to keep you as a returning customer because that's where the money is. You might be one of those women who's gone backwards and forwards to slimming clubs. Maybe you've stuck with the same one because 'it works'. Maybe you've tried lots of different ones. Whatever you're doing, if it worked, you probably wouldn't need to come back. Now I'm not saying it's all about the slimming club because a lot of the reason we can't lose weight is to do with our own mindset and the diet messages that we've absorbed over a long period of time, but slimming clubs definitely have a part to play in the confusion that women feel about their weight loss.

We don't need to make food into points. We don't need to label food as sinful. We don't need to demonise any type of food.

So, what is the answer? Is there an answer? Yes, there's an answer! The answer is to ditch the BS and give something new a try, something that is probably going to feel uncomfortable to start with because you don't think it's going to work. It's going to seem a lot easier than what you've been doing. You're still going to be able to have a life. Imagine that, losing weight and having a life, who knew the two things could go together?

Why W.E.I.G.H.T?

Let's face it, not many of us enjoy being on the dieting treadmill, we would much rather be living our lives knowing that we won't put on oodles of weight that we've constantly got to keep shifting every time someone has a birthday, there's a holiday, or it's Christmas or the cat passes its degree. The ideal solution is to find something that allows you to continue living your life whilst you work on your weight loss. Something that seems so simple that you barely even notice you're doing it. Of course, there are going to be compromises, there's going to need to be change, but the way that we do that, the way that we make this work is to do things differently. Real success comes down to a mindset change. Unless you change your way of thinking you will probably always find yourself back at square one. I've worked with plenty of women who refuse to believe that there might be a different way and they're constantly drawn back to their old patterns of avoiding carbohydrates, doing hours of cardio etc., all the things that aren't actually serving them. I don't blame these women at all for the way that they feel and think, because it is really hard to change that mind-set. I know because I was trapped in it for a long time thinking that unless I was starving myself to try to be skinny that nothing else was going to work. I would avoid foods that I wanted to eat because I thought I 'couldn't' eat them and then binge them in a really unhealthy way. I was miserable when I went out to eat because I was worried about what I could and couldn't choose on the menu in case it made me fat.

So, what led me to come up with my W.E.I.G.H.T method of weight loss? Well, firstly, having been trapped in a cycle of disordered eating, for many years; when I had my daughter, I no longer wanted to be like that. I didn't want her to grow up a slave to the diet industry, a slave to wanting to lose weight all the time, a slave to being permanently unhappy with herself. I didn't want her to be weighing herself every day and having that stupid piece of machinery deciding whether she was going to be in a good mood or not. I also entered a career in the fitness industry and worked with lots of women who were also following similar crazy ideas and flogging themselves to death for very little result. I'd see them enthusiastically starting their plan, only to tail off after a couple of weeks because it was just unsustainable, too hard to stick to and didn't fit their lifestyle, making them miserable in the process. They might have been unhappy about their weight but the way they were trying to lose weight was making them more miserable. Once the enthusiasm waned and the misery set in, I wouldn't see them for a few months, and then they'd be back again with the same goal in mind, but maybe having put on even more weight. They had tried lots of different things but would be convinced that following the same path was the answer. All of this led me to create something that would help women lose weight in a healthy way and focus more on keeping the weight off long term rather than just losing weight in the short term.

Chapter Two

The good news is that I have created the solution with my W.E.I.G.H.T framework. My W.E.I.G.H.T framework helps you to lose weight and keep it off for life while still living your life without misery or restriction.

WEIGHT stands for:

Weed out the BS

Enjoy your food again

Individualise your plan

Get moving

Habits

The 4 Ts

Why this? It's a simple process, but one that treats you as an individual which means it will be the perfect match for you. No complicated meal plans or points to count and no foods are demonised!

How will my W.E.I.G.H.T framework help you achieve this?

Firstly, we're going to weed out the BS starting with all those diet myths that you've absorbed over your lifetime. We're going to separate the fact from the myth and set you on a lighter path and one that's way simpler to understand and get you to your actual goals. We'll be looking at your mindset and largely this will relate back to those diet myths that you've absorbed. These have played with our minds about food, about exercise, about our bodies and left us confused; not knowing where to turn. This step is an incredibly important one in ensuring that you can keep the weight off. Unless you think about your mindset, and make those necessary changes, you will always find yourself ending up back at square one, maybe even further back than you were originally. We don't want that anymore. We want to keep moving forward. We want to spend less time worrying about dieting and more time enjoying our lives.

We're going to work on a healthier mindset. One that allows us to look at food and lifestyle in a different way. From there, we're going to delve a bit deeper looking at our own limiting beliefs. These are things that we tell ourselves every day that sometimes don't have any foundation anymore. They might have been things we heard about ourselves as a child or as a teenager and again, we've absorbed those messages and still carry them around with us. When it comes to weight loss, these limiting beliefs can really hold us back as we start to think of ourselves as failures or 'I'm just always going to be this way'. Looking at the limiting beliefs that we have, working through them and understanding that some of them might not apply anymore and start to turn those limiting beliefs into something more positive, that keeps us moving forward.

After we've dealt with all that crap we've been carrying around, we're going to move on to our relationship with food. Enjoying your food again is going to be a vital part of your weight loss success. I know you may think this sounds counterproductive - surely I'm meant to be enjoying my food less if I'm going to get any real improvements from my weight loss programme? It's the relationship we have with food that's going to be key to your success. We're going to look at the thoughts and feelings we have around food. Are there really good and bad foods? Does the type of food we eat matter?

Next, we'll identify your non-negotiables. What you are prepared to compromise on and what you are absolutely not willing to give up is a really important part of individualising your weight loss plan and making it work for you.

We'll look at how to make eating for weight loss as simple as possible so that it can EASILY fit into your busy lifestyle. As a woman we often have several plates spinning all at one time and the last thing we need to be presented with is a healthy recipe that takes three hours to prepare and an overnight cook - that's never going to lead to success. The easier we make it the better it will be.

Lastly, we'll be working on planning. Planning is **key** for success in most areas of our lives and losing weight and keeping it off is no different. We will start to put together a meal plan that works for you. Thinking about your working hours, whether you're driving the kids to club, taking parents to hospital appointments or trying to de-worm the cat or just make life simpler. Once you realise how easy it is to plan ahead and what a difference that makes, it will become second nature to you and form the basis of your weekly diet. Individualising your plan is what sets this weight loss framework apart from the others. You are not the same as Brenda from accounts, Babs from down the road or Jenny who drinks in your local! You're all very different and therefore a one size fits all plan is not the answer. Just because Brenda in accounts decided to give up bread, pasta, potatoes and joy, doesn't mean that you should. Just because Susan works out for two hours a day and cries for the other 22 does not mean that you should. Just because Jenny's miserably staring into her meal replacement shake twice a day does not mean you should.

We're going to take all the things that we've already worked on; looking at your lifestyle; what your non-negotiables are; what's going on for you. How will this weight loss plan fit into your lifestyle so it is simple and doesn't become another job to add to the to do list. From there, we will make the plan work around you. Maybe there are days when you have a busy schedule and preparing a meal is a no go. How can we make that day as stress free as possible for you so that you are able to stay on track and still fulfil everything that you've got in your diary that day?

Get moving. In this chapter we'll be looking at why movement is important. And how it can help boost your weight loss results. We will demystify the difference between movement and exercise and how much you should be doing of each in order to get the best results. So many of us live sedentary lifestyles these days, desk jobs, hours on the sofa scrolling, streaming boxsets, that our movement and level of activity has really decreased. You'll be surprised how just making some simple changes in this area can really help move you towards your target a lot quicker than you anticipated. Don't stress about this. It doesn't have to be strenuous. Again it's about picking out your non-negotiables - what are you prepared to do in terms of movement? And what are you not prepared to do? Just because your friend Sarah likes to bang out 50 burpees until she vomits every morning does not mean that is what you need to be doing! (Disclaimer I would not recommend this as a healthy way to get moving straight away).

Habits are the next step to succeeding in your weight loss plan. Often the reason we've put on weight is because we've picked up some bad habits. We didn't pick these up immediately. We didn't eat five chocolate bars one day and then start eating five chocolate bars every day. It built up over time. And the exact same happens when we're trying to instil good habits. We'll be looking at what habits you need to start working on and how they can easily slot into your lifestyle. We'll be looking at what difference this will make to your weight loss journey and how to effectively implement habits to get the best results.

Lastly, I'll be asking you to take a pretty big step in most of our minds and that is to trust yourself. Years of dieting and diet messages can make us lose trust in ourselves. We lose confidence in our ability to know when we should stop eating; fail to understand when we're hungry and to know what actual portion sizes should look like. Unless we're being told what to do by a diet company or slimming club, we feel out of our depth.

How do I know when to eat, should I eat after six? Only eat between the hours of 10 and six, do I fast for 12 hours? When do I have my protein shake, when do I have my meal replacement shake? Should I drink water in case I'm not really hungry but just thirsty? With all these things running through our heads, and I'm sure there's way more than those few that I've mentioned, diets really play with our minds and our confidence. You **do** know what to do. You **do** have all the skills that you need in order to lose weight, but it really comes back to believing in ourselves and this final chapter will help you do that!

Now let's get down to the nitty gritty!

Chapter Three - Weed Out The BS

Why is this chapter important? Because, as women we're fed so many diets and so much diet advice, telling us what we should and shouldn't be eating, when we should and shouldn't be eating and then changing it all again. So unless we cut through all this noise and get to the crux of the matter we're not going to be able to move forward. A lot of the stuff you're being told is simply to sell you something, to hook you in so that you keep buying a product or a service and to make you feel unable to carry on unless you buy into these things. Most of these diet plans and fads and services don't want you to succeed because if you succeed, then they lose your money.

As I've said most of us don't want to lose weight, we want to *lose weight and keep it off*. Most of what we're sold is solely about losing weight in the short term, to give quick results, but not helping us to sustain it. And that's where it's going wrong.

This chapter is all about cutting through all that stuff, figuring out what is right and what isn't. What's going to help you the most to succeed and what is going to hold you back. We're going to start by looking at some diet myths breaking them down and getting really honest about what's really going on.

Myth number one: You must stop eating all your favourite foods in order to lose weight.

This whole concept of giving up all the foods that you love is just ridiculous. Food is food regardless of whether it's crisps, broccoli, potatoes, chocolate, it's all just food. You could eat chocolate all day long and lose weight as long as you don't go over your calorie allowance, whatever that may be for you. The idea that you have to give up all the foods that you love, which normally end up being the ones that might be more calorific or more fatty, because let's face it, those things taste nice, usually leads us to give up with our weight loss plans. It becomes impossible to stick to something if we don't feel we can have those foods that we genuinely enjoy that make us feel like we're having something special. There's absolutely no need to give up any of your favourite foods in order to lose weight; your diet might just need some balance and compromise, but you do not have to give them up. This is one idea you will hopefully end up losing by reading this book.

Myth number two: What you weigh is the most important factor in your weight loss plan.

A huge myth! Our weight fluctuates on a daily, sometimes even hourly basis. I could weigh myself in the morning and be a completely different weight at night. I could weigh myself on Monday and be a completely different weight on the Tuesday. There are so many factors involved in what you weigh, water weight, muscle, bone, whether you've been to toilet... The list goes on! And the number on the scale is not always a true measurement of weight loss or gain.

Whilst we're on this topic, let's delve a little bit deeper. When we say weight loss, most of us really want fat loss. It's fat loss that makes the most difference to how we look. So when we are thinking weight loss what we want to make sure is that we are losing fat and not just muscle and water.

I used to find that stepping on the scales could change my whole day. If I stepped on the scales and the number wasn't something I was hoping to see it would change my mood, it would change how I perceived myself, how I looked at my body. I could have been feeling absolutely fine before stepping on the scales but as soon as that number didn't tell me what I wanted, I'd have a whole completely different mindset for the day ahead.

Now, I totally get why people want to use the scales as a measurement of how well they're doing. Again, it comes down to something we've been told our entire lives, this is the way we should be measuring our progress. Slimming clubs usually use scales to measure your progress and you'll often find in that first week, or the first few weeks, you might lose an awful lot of weight on the scales. Largely, this is down to losing water and muscle mass. We do not want to be losing muscle mass as this is actually counterproductive to us losing fat but for slimming clubs, this works really well because you have massive weight loss to start with and it spurs you on and keeps you going back to the club. Obviously, anything that incentivises you to get going is great but only if it ends up being a true reflection of your progress. Also, the more weight we lose the harder it becomes to lose even more weight, which again can become totally demoralising.

Myth number three: You have to be miserable in order to lose weight.

You absolutely do not need to feel miserable during your weight loss plan. Usually this ties in with weight loss myth one - having to cut out all our favourite foods. So why do we feel miserable when we're trying to lose weight? Because we give up our favourite foods and go to extremes with our food plan. We might even add in some exercise that we hate in order to boost our weight loss results. This in turn is obviously going to make us miserable and we're no longer enjoying the journey, and I'm sure we can agree that weight loss can be a long journey sometimes. That's why getting a good balance on eating foods that you love and foods that support your weight loss but are still tasty and enjoyable, alongside finding ways to move that make you feel good, and fit your lifestyle, is imperative to your success. If you are on a weight loss plan and you feel miserable, I advise you to stop doing it immediately. Life is way too short to feel like that!

Myth number four: Bread is your enemy if you're trying to lose weight.

Now some people might say I am slightly obsessed with bread. But I'm not really, I just feel sorry for it because it gets a hard rap. There's a lot of breadism out there and we're not having it. Now, of course, if you eat bread or any other carbohydrate in excessive amounts, taking you over the number of calories that you need, then you're going to put on weight, but the same would happen if you overeat vegetables or salad!

We just need to think about how we eat them and eat them in the right portions so we can still enjoy them without them hindering our weight loss success. You may find as you get older that eating a lot of carbohydrates doesn't serve you well anymore, but that doesn't mean that you need to cut them out altogether.

Myth number five: You need to figure out your macronutrients in order to succeed with your weight loss plan.

Now macronutrients have been a buzzword for a long time now. And I often see women who haven't even nailed the basics of healthy eating and weight loss, worrying about how many grams of carbohydrates, protein, and fats they're having. Carbohydrate, proteins and fats are basically known collectively as your macronutrients.

When you're starting out on your weight loss plan, we want to keep things as simple as possible. We need you to be able to do this. And if you're constantly worrying about whether you've eaten 35 or 40 grams of carbohydrates, it's going to get complicated and you're going to get overwhelmed. Then what happens? You end up back at that point where you give up because it's too much.

Myth number six: Calories don't count on a weight loss plan.

Now, you might think, 'yes, stupid, that is obviously a myth. Every diet I've ever done is about calories.' But there is an idea bandied about that calories aren't important when you're trying to lose weight. Sorry to say calories are important because if you're overeating and taking in too many calories, you are going to gain weight, simple as that! However, it doesn't mean that you must live a life of calorie counting for evermore in order to stay at your ideal weight or to lose weight. There's lots of other ways that you can figure out how to reduce your calories without inputting them into an app or figuring out on a bit of a piece of paper.

Myth number seven: You should eat at certain times in order to optimise weight loss.

It doesn't matter when you eat. You can eat after 6pm! You can eat at midnight if you want to. You don't have to eat every four hours or so many times a day. What it comes down to is how many calories you're eating and whether you're eating more than you need.

I could probably write a whole book on weight loss myths alone and maybe I will one day just for the hell of it but the important thing is that we look at these ideas that we've been fed and we see how these might be hindering us more than helping us. It's not helpful for us to be worrying about whether we eat after 6pm, whether we had an extra piece of bread on Tuesday or to be crying in the cake aisle at the supermarket because you missed cake so much.

What's important is that we get over these myths, to accept that they are myths. This can take some work because we're used to living by these rules and to move away from them can seem scary. Moving out of our comfort zone can feel scary and it's no different when it comes to weight loss. A lot of women are brainwashed when it comes to weight loss and diets. You're not alone in that and most of the time we don't even realise it because we're absorbing this information all the time. Hopefully seeing some of these weight loss myths and picking out the ones that you have been led to believe and have been basing your weight loss plan around, can help you start to move toward a new way of thinking.

Now, obviously, you can probably think of some other diet advice or guidance you've been given that you're not sure is true, but I thought I'd focus on some of the top few, the ones that seem to bother women the most, the myths that seem to feature most often in the minds of women who are trying to lose weight.

What's next in weeding out the BS when it comes to weight loss? Mindset! This ties in nicely with those weight loss myths that we've just discussed. Some of you have probably read those weight loss myths and are thinking, 'Oh, I dunno, I ate that time after 6pm one night and the next day I weighed more.' 'I had a takeaway two months ago and then at the next weigh in I was over my target weight.'

'Jane in accounts said she once ate a sandwich and the next day she was 2 stone heavier.'

All of these things, or at least some of these or similar thoughts are going through your head right now. 'Who is this woman telling us these things aren't true? These are the things we've relied on for the past 20, 30 maybe even 40 years! They must be true. Everyone knows that.' And this is where your **mindset** really comes into its own. Changing your mindset is so important. We touched on it earlier in the book, how mindset is the key to success. You can make all the food changes you like, you can add in more movement, but if your mindset is still back where you were before, you're always going to come to a certain point and get stuck and that's what we need to change. If you're always getting stuck, you're never going to move forward to the point where you're *actually* able to keep the weight off. You do know how to keep the weight off, but the diet industry has made you feel that you don't know, you don't trust yourself anymore and you think it doesn't matter because there will always be a quick fix to turn to!

We need to get you through the anxiety of letting go of these incorrect ideals that you've held on to. Ultimately all these myths have taught you are that you are not able to make progress by yourself. You can't be trusted around food. You can't be trusted to make good decisions about your eating habits. And this leads to a total lack of confidence in yourself.

We need to change the all or nothing mindset that you probably have if you want to lose weight and the thinking that success and misery go hand in hand. We need to change the mindset that the quick fix is the answer and start to embrace the fact that a slower and more sustainable process is the one that's going to get you from sad to happy.

Losing weight is a journey! It's about a lifestyle and this is going to be your **new** mindset, thinking about the things that you are prepared to change, that you can do for the rest of your life. Now, I know that sounds scary! Whaaaat? A lifetime?? I'm not ready for that. Don't think like that, because yes, it's a lifetime commitment, but one that will suit you and your lifestyle. It doesn't mean that you're never going to be able to eat a takeaway again, or your favourite chocolate bar or cheese, (because no one should have to give cheese up)! If having a takeaway on a Friday night with your family is important to you then giving it up in the short term in order to lose weight is not going to help you in the long term. We need to make sure that takeaway is included in your individual plan. How you are going to make that work in terms of your weight loss and your weight loss maintenance, which as I keep harping on about, is the important bit.

You know you can lose weight; after all, you've probably done this time and time again! The part you're probably struggling with is keeping it off. This is where you can make changes that don't need too much effort that you can stick to easily until these changes become part of your daily habits.

Let look at an example of an easy habit you can probably repeat for life that will benefit your weight loss. Sugar in your hot drinks! Reducing the amount of sugar you have in your hot drinks is probably something that you can do for the rest of your life because you're not giving up the sugar if you don't want to, but by reducing it, you are automatically cutting calories. And if you're like me and drink tea like it's going out of fashion, then you might be consuming quite a lot of sugar during the day!

Another thing we need to do as part of our whole weeding activity is to cut our own self-limiting beliefs. Now many of these beliefs we're often carrying around with us from childhood or our younger years. Statements such as 'oh, she's always so loud' which either makes us louder or causes us to shrink into the background because we're worried that we're going to be too much for people. When it comes to weight loss, we might have been told things like 'she was always a big eater', 'she flits from thing to thing all the time' and I'm sure you can think of statements that you've heard about yourself time and time again. We absorb this information, and it can affect how we go about our life. If we constantly hear the same things around food, for example, having a big appetite or never turning down food this could have a knock-on effect, leading you to eat in secret or emotional eating through guilt. It might cause you to be in denial, telling yourself, and others, 'I hardly eat anything at all and I still can't lose weight', when really you're not counting the things that you are eating in secret for fear of that judgement and because you've taken on that limiting belief.

We can switch our mindset around those self-limiting beliefs and turn them into something more positive, something that allows us to succeed. So instead of 'oh, she's got such a big appetite', how about 'she really loves food and she's always got such healthy meals?' You know, you can eat a lot of food if you're picking the right foods to eat. So therefore, having a big appetite wouldn't be a problem at all. If you've been told that you always flit from thing to thing all that means is that with this weight loss process that I'm suggesting to you, you're going to be willing to try it which is a way more positive way to frame this. These self-limiting beliefs can really affect us and hold us back and we want to get rid of them so we can move forward. Remember that you're the only person who has control over the steps you take to move forward.

Where would you be now if you'd started a more positive approach to your weight loss five years ago? Would you be out living your best life without worrying about whether you had potatoes at that restaurant on Friday? Or stepping on the scales every morning to check you haven't gained half a pound?

Stop letting these beliefs hold you back. Again, it's not going to be easy work. We've all got things that we have to work through that are difficult and sometimes uncomfortable but once we do it, we can really move ourselves forward into a whole new space

And the only one living your life is you, if other people have those beliefs about you, who's to say that they're true? Who's to say a belief that someone had about you as a child, is the same now you're an adult? You've grown, you've evolved and you can keep on growing and evolving.

Let's cut this BS and take those strides forward towards our goals.

So, in summary, what is the stuff that works?

Look at any diet myths that you've absorbed and think about whether they've truly helped you in the past, not just in the short term, but in the long term. I'm guessing probably not, as you're reading this book and I'm going to suggest that probably most of you are here because you've tried things and they haven't worked in the past! Don't worry you're not alone.

Forget the myths you've been told, all you need to worry about is whether you are consuming more calories than you are burning! It doesn't matter what other weight loss spin anyone is putting on it that is the crux of the matter.

Secondly, work on your mindset and how you feel about those diet myths and weight loss in general, if you've got a negative view of it and you feel it's a restrictive and miserable thing to do; this could be affecting your success.

Think about why it's important to you to lose weight? What's life going to look like when you've lost the weight that you hope to lose?

Have you lost weight before and found that you weren't that happy when you got to the weight you thought you should be? What's going to be different if you lose the weight and keep it off?

A large part of working on your mindset is really thinking about the why? It needs to be important enough to you to keep you going.

Why W.E.I.G.H.T?

Takeaways!

1. What diet messages have you absorbed over the years? Jot them down below and reflect on whether they have helped you to lose weight ***and keep it off!***
2. What elements of your mindset do you need to work on? What's holding you back?
3. What's your why? Why is this important to you?
4. What changes can you start to make immediately? Think small and doable, not hard and restrictive.

<table>
<tr><td>Diet messages I have absorbed: -</td></tr>
<tr><td>1.</td></tr>
<tr><td>2.</td></tr>
<tr><td>3.</td></tr>
<tr><td>4.</td></tr>
<tr><td>5.</td></tr>
</table>

<table>
<tr><td>What parts of my mind-set do I need to work on first?</td></tr>
<tr><td>1.</td></tr>
<tr><td>2.</td></tr>
<tr><td>3.</td></tr>
</table>

What's my why? Why is this so important to me?

What one change could I start making today?

Chapter Four - Enjoy your food again

The thing with more traditional dieting is that it can actually take away the enjoyment of your food because it either involves so much planning and thought, or because it doesn't allow you to eat a wide variety of foods while giving negative labels to some of the foods that you do enjoy. The problem with this is that it can lead to an unsustainable way of eating and a very disordered way of thinking about food.

How do we start to enjoy our food again whilst still losing weight and keeping it off for life? First, we need to ditch the idea that some foods are good and bad. How often have you heard yourself saying 'oh, I can't eat that food, it's bad for me'. Or even worse, you found yourself saying 'I was bad last night because I ate x' or 'I've had a really bad week'. This is where that disordered thinking about food comes into play. We've picked up those messages through diets we've tried in the past and they've seeped into every area of our life so now we do associate foods as being good or bad. Even worse, we associate ourselves with being good or bad depending on what we've eaten that day. What we need to do is ditch this mentality because there is no good and bad! There are just some foods that you should eat more of and some foods that you can still enjoy, but maybe a little bit less than you might be right now. For example, cake, chocolate and crisps. There's nothing wrong with those foods, it's just that if we eat them in huge amounts, plus all our other food that we're consuming, of course we're going to put on weight. But if we cut those foods out, when we do enjoy them sometimes and want to be able to eat them, we just end up either secretly bingeing on them or coming off our diet altogether and just going back to square one. Or we end up walking around in a permanent fog of misery because we spend hours down the cake aisle drooling at the things that we can't have.

The idea of good and bad whether you're associating it with food or yourself is not conducive to moving forward with your weight loss goals.

Why W.E.I.G.H.T?

Anything that makes us feel bad about ourselves is not going to help us to succeed. As I mentioned before, we can absolutely eat whatever we want as long as we're eating it in the right amounts. You could live off cake and lose weight if you're eating it in the right amount. You might not be at your healthiest but you could still lose weight. Ideally though, we want to be losing weight and maintaining our health because our health is way more important than what size jeans we're getting into. But the good news is we can do both! Woohoo! We can be healthy; we can lose weight and even better we can get to enjoy foods that we like!

How do you stop thinking of foods and yourself as good and bad when it's so ingrained? Remember that anything that you eat in abundance can potentially lead you to gain weight, so therefore all foods are equal in that capacity. A lot of the idea of some foods being fat burning or super foods is purely a marketing ploy in order to get you to buy them and usually these foods have a higher price attached to them.

You need to remember that what you thought was a bad food or a good food a year ago is probably the opposite now because the diet industry has changed its mind about what you should and shouldn't eat. What we need to do is to start thinking of food as food. Some food we eat because it serves a purpose in terms of providing us with the minerals and vitamins that we need to give us energy, fibre, protein and good fats. We eat these foods because they are a better choice for us for the majority of the time.

Sometimes we might associate those foods with being boring or not tasting very nice, but it certainly doesn't have to be that way. There are simple ways to spice up your salads and boujee your broccoli! Then there are some foods that we eat because they taste nice or because they're associated with happy occasions such as cake on birthdays, chocolate when we're at the cinema, take away while we watch a movie. Those foods are just as valid in our life as all the other foods that we're choosing to eat but we just have to think a bit more about how often we eat them. Remember, what we're doing here is trying to make changes that we can adhere to for the rest of our lives. So if we're saying that we're going to cut out all the things like cake and takeaways, chances are we're not going to stick to that forever because there's always going to be someone's birthday or a movie night or takeaway with the girls. We must learn how to incorporate those things into our diet without them leading to us going on a total spiral!

The second thing is to recognise that we are not good or bad for eating or not eating certain foods. Just because Brenda at work always declines the Friday cake does not make her any better than you and vice versa. There might be a million reasons why Brenda's declining Friday cake. She might have cake Monday to Thursday, but you just don't know about that.

One of the best ways to separate yourself from being good or bad is to accept that you do have a choice over what you eat all the time.

By recognising that choosing to have cake on a Friday because you enjoy it doesn't mean that you're undoing all the good work you've done with your healthy eating. This allows you to enjoy the cake and continue with your day without spending the rest of it feeling guilt ridden and needing to confess to anyone who will listen how bad you've been! This 'I'm a good or bad person' mentality when it comes to food doesn't serve us in achieving our weight loss goals.

If you think about choosing foods on the basis that you're doing the best thing for you, your body and your health means you're doing it from a position of loving yourself. If your frame of mind is 'I'm a bad person because I ate cake yesterday, or I had a chocolate bar on the way home from work' that's all coming from a place of not loving yourself. Realistically, we don't put much effort into things we hate or dislike (unless we're getting paid lol)! We put much more effort into things we love.

Then we need to think about identifying our non-negotiables. As I said we tend to go quite extreme when we go on a diet, cutting out all those foods that we associate as being bad, but we actually like to eat. Now if there's certain things that you're not that bothered about giving up, for example maybe you don't need a packet of crisps every day for lunch, maybe you don't need a chocolate bar at three o'clock every day – if you're happy to lose those things, that's great. But if you absolutely look forward to that chocolate bar at three o'clock in the afternoon when you have your cup of tea, then factor that into your plan, acknowledge that you're not prepared to give that up. People that know me will know that one of my non-negotiables is that I will always have two chocolate biscuits every day. It's a part of my diet because I don't want to give up chocolate biscuits. I don't have to eat chocolate biscuits every day, sometimes I don't, but the very fact that I know that I can because I've allowed for it within my eating plan and my lifestyle gives me that freedom to have it without that feeling of guilt. If I didn't do that and I had the chocolate biscuits, I might end up in that cycle of guilt leading to me eating all the chocolate biscuits because I feel bad about myself, wondering what's the point and bingeing. Knowing that I can have these things in my diet sometimes means that I actually don't need them and I won't eat them after all, but just knowing you can have them makes a whole heap of difference to reaching your targets.

Maybe there are other things that you can negotiate with yourself, for example, reducing the amount of sugars you have in your tea; reducing the amount of milky coffees you drink a day; substituting calorie laden soft drinks for the sugar free versions; there will always be something that you can compromise on without having to give everything up. The non-negotiables are really important because it identifies what's important to you as an individual rather than what a diet plan is telling you that you need to do. We're all different! What I might consider important in my diet is completely different from you. You might not give a monkeys about whether you have chocolate biscuits or not, but you might feel really strongly about having crisps with your lunch. That's fine. We've all got things that we identify as important to us.

Now obviously there is going to have to be some element of compromise. If you say that your non-negotiables are basically everything, then we're not really going to move forward, but identifying some foods that we are not prepared to give up completely allows us to factor that in when we build our individual weight loss plans. Once we've identified the things that we're not so happy to cut out of our diet or reduce in our diet, we can look at the things that we can change from there because we've already figured out what's important to us. I think once you start to do your individual plan and see what you can still eat whilst still losing weight and keeping it off, you'll feel a lot of the stress of dieting, leave you!

Thirdly, keep it super simple! We are much more likely to do something that's easy then do something that's complicated and hard. Especially, as let's face it; we are all busy these days! What does keeping it super simple look like? Well again, it looks at you as an individual. What does life look like on a day to day or weekly basis for you? What days are busy for you? What days might you need to think about a bit more than others? Making things simpler for you, for example, would prepping your lunches help you be more organised in the morning and feel less rushed? Maybe having some healthy choice ready meals in at home means that on a particularly busy day you can come in and instantly throw something in the oven while you shower and get your PJs on. Feeling stressed about your weight loss plan is counterintuitive. Stress can be a predominant factor in why we can struggle to lose weight and if we're thinking about doing this for the rest of our lives the last thing we want is for it to stress us out! We want it to be as easy as possible - slipping into our lifestyle as easily as a random stranger might slip into our DMS on Instagram!

Keeping it super simple also involves thinking about cooking from scratch! You'll be pleased to know it doesn't need to be a 13-page recipe with 200 ingredients that means you travelling to a specialty shop in a town 30 miles away to purchase. We can cook good food at home from scratch without it being complicated, without involving lots of ingredients at huge cost and hours in the kitchen. If that's your bag, fine! If you're able to and have the time to create wonderful healthy meals, then go for it. We'll all sit here and just silently seethe with jealousy that you've got the skills to produce something magical and fresh from the latest series of MasterChef, but whatever your skills are, and whatever your time factor, cooking from scratch does not need to be complicated. There are loads of ways that you can make salmon and chicken and Quorn more varied and exciting to eat without spending a huge amount of time on it.

Moving forward, what do we need to do? We need to spend some time working on that good and bad mentality. Try listening to yourself so that when you hear yourself using terms such as good or bad to refer to yourself, you take a minute and try to change that language and do the same when you're talking about foods.

Write down what your non-negotiables are. Have a think about it. You don't need to do this in a rush. You can do it over a week or two. What's important to you to include in your diet? Write these down so that you have them ready when you come to do your individual plan.

Think about what's going to make it super simple for you to stick to your plan when you get it. Is it going to be having a meal plan for the week? Is it going to be prepping your lunches? What is it that you're not doing right now that causes you stress when it comes to losing weight and managing your food? Getting these things in place will really help you move forward and smash those weight loss goals.

Takeaways

1. Do you describe yourself or foods as good or bad? How does using these labels make you feel and does it get the results you want? Try being more aware of the language you are using.
2. What are your non-negotiables? Decide these so you know what you are and are not prepared to give up.
3. Don't overcomplicate it! The simpler you make things the better – remember it's better to do things bit by bit than go all in and give up!

What are your non-negotiables when it comes to food?

Chapter Five – Individualise your plan

The important part of this weight loss programme is the individualisation. You've tried one size fits all diet plans before and they haven't worked.

Picking a diet plan/weight loss plan/fat loss plan that works for you is going to be way more effective in getting the results you want. Why? Because it's going to fit everything you need it to, it's going to work with your lifestyle. That means it's going to be easier to stick to and you'll be able to make it fit without really noticing much significant change, except in your weight loss of course!

Where do we start? You need to think about where you are now. It's really important that you do this part of the work because if you don't know your starting point how can you make the right decisions about what to do in order to move forward? Most of us skip this step when we think about losing weight. We don't pay attention to what our diet currently looks like, how much we're eating; how much we're moving; what other things are going on in our life, we just go straight in making changes to our food and possibly our exercise. As I've said before, often the changes can be quite dramatic and feel quite restrictive and that's why it doesn't work. Think about it this way, if you don't know where you are now, and you don't know how much you're eating and you just decide to slash all your food intake down to about 1000 calories, the results are you're hungry, you're miserable and soon you're giving up because it's too hard to stick to. What you didn't realise is that you were actually consuming 3000 calories a day, you've knocked 2000 calories off, no wonder you're starving.

If you'd done the work and realised where you were starting from you would have known the adjustments to make. Just to add as a disclaimer, I don't think you should be on a 1000 calorie diet I was just using that as an example. Take a good honest look at where you are now. How much food are you eating? It's a good idea to keep a food diary or take photos of everything that you eat so you can see it visually. (A visual food diary can often be really powerful). From that you can look and decide what changes you can make. It doesn't have to be about counting calories necessarily it can just be about making reductions and cutting certain things out. For example, say you always get up in the morning and have three slices of buttery toast, two scrambled eggs, followed by a full bowl of cereal and three coffees with two sugars in each you might think about cutting that down, so still have your scrambled eggs but on two pieces or one piece of toast. Reduce the amount of butter you have. Go down to one sugar in your coffee and halve the amount of cereal that you're having in the morning. You're still having the same breakfast as you had before, but just on a smaller scale without any dramatic calorie reductions. Making small changes like that can make a huge difference but you can't make those changes if you haven't figured out what you were doing in the first place. And let's be honest, if most of us are asked about what we eat we can often be found guilty of a little white lie sometimes!

This is where this plan is different as most weight loss plans don't consider your starting point. It's much easier to work with where you are now than to work with where you want to be in the future.

When you're looking at where you are now you can look at how much movement you're doing. Think about how much time you're sitting down throughout the day and from there you can think about how much more movement you can add in. Have you got time to exercise? Have you got time to go for a walk? If you're not doing any sort of movement at the moment suddenly deciding that you're going to run five kilometres three times a week is probably going to be unachievable and end up making you feel pretty crappy when you can't do it. If you're not moving much why not decide to start walking for 10 minutes every other day. It's more achievable. It doesn't take up too much of your time. Again, it's not too much of a shock to the system from what you've already been doing. You're more likely to stick to it and increase your activity from there.

Hopefully you can see that looking at where you are starting from is so important to the outcome.

Looking at your starting point may also include examining some of those barriers and obstacles to achieving your goals. For example, maybe having children is a bit of a barrier if you don't have childcare to allow you to go out and exercise. Maybe you do shift work and you find that a barrier when it comes to eating healthy meals and cooking food from scratch. Looking at all those things allows you to see exactly what the big picture is - what's really going on and from there it's so much easier to create solutions, and more importantly solutions that work for you.

The next step is back to those non-negotiables that we've already spoken about. There's no point putting anything in your plan that you're not actually prepared to do and prepared to do in the long term. You might be prepared to do it in the first week or the first day or the first hour but if you're not prepared to do it long term, there's absolutely no point including it. For example, if you're going to cut out pasta, but actually you love pasta the plan is just not going to work for you. Keep the pasta in and think about your portions. But there's no point making promises to yourself that you know you're not going to keep.

Choosing our non-negotiables allows us to make room for those things that we enjoy eating and that are important to us - that take away with the family; the meal out with the girls at the end of the month; those two chocolate biscuits you're dunking at the end of the day… Maybe that's just me!

The same applies with the exercise side of your non-negotiables. Thinking again about the example of the five-kilometre run I mentioned earlier, there's no point putting that in your plan if you hate running and it's therefore unlikely that you're going to be able to stick to it. Find something that you enjoy or can at least tolerate and do that instead. Remember, we're thinking of a lifelong plan, not a quick fix, and that's what makes this successful.

Be realistic. We've touched on this already when we spoke about our non-negotiables it's not realistic to think that you're going to exercise every day. It's not realistic to expect that you're never going to eat the things that you've said you're not going to eat. It's not realistic that you're going to be perfect. If we set those challenges and goals that are unachievable, we end up with that feeling of failure and that leads us to go back into that diet cycle that we're trying to get out of. We eat, we feel bad because we've eaten so we eat more and the cycle continues. If we're realistic with ourselves, if we accept that, 'you know what; I know I'm not going to be perfect. I know I'm not going to eat the whole grain rice and the salad and the vegetables all the time. I know that sometimes yeah, I'm going to go out to eat, I'm going to have a few drinks, I'm going to have a takeaway, I'm going to eat more chocolate than I intended to'. If you accept that's going to happen then it's more likely that you will be able to move on instead of harbouring it, deep down in your soul and letting it ruin your life for the next 10 years before you start your diet again!

Thinking about your non-negotiables, be realistic about what you will and won't do in terms of food and exercise. If you hate the gym signing up for a year's membership at your local gym is not going to be the answer to your weight loss. If you hate kale starting the kale and rice diet is not going to be ideal either.

Time! Be realistic in terms of what time you have in the day, what time you have in the week. When is it realistic that you're going to be able to get your movement in, when is it realistic that you're going to be able to cook meals, when is it realistic you're going to be able to prep lunches? If like me you're not that keen on getting out of bed very early, plotting in 6am workouts are probably not the answer. It's not realistic so you're not going to keep it up – I know I don't! Maybe lunchtime or an evening suits you better. It's important to be honest with yourself. Individualising your plan is in no way a judgement of your choices. For you to succeed, they need to be your choices.

We also need to understand that we will need to compromise if we're going to lose weight. I much prefer the word 'compromise' to 'sacrifice'. Sad as it may be, there are going to be times where you're going to have to turn down certain food items or you can't have the whole Victoria sponge but without this compromise, you're not going to move forward and thinking about it in terms of a compromise still means you've got a choice. Sacrifice indicates that choice is taken away from you. If we talk about compromise, it means that we're always in control of the choices that we make. This is really empowering and feeling empowered is much more likely to allow us to succeed than if we feel that we don't have any control.

Lastly, let's begin thinking about what you can start today! Building a plan is not thinking what it might look like five years from now. Often thinking too far ahead trips us up because when we don't get there, we become disheartened and give up. Recognising this cycle of dieting will help you to quickly veer away from that path if you start heading down it. If we think in the short term - what one thing can I start doing today? – We are more likely to achieve it and feel motivated to continue. That one thing could be reducing the amount of sugar you have in your hot drinks, reducing the amount of full fat lattes you grab on the way to work or increasing your fruit and veg or water intake. Whatever that one thing is you feel you can get started with today. And it doesn't need to be overwhelming - you can aim to drink water for at least three days of the week, you can aim to reduce your sugar for at least one day a week, you can choose that you might only have crisps with your lunch every other day. It doesn't have to be all or nothing. You can always build up once you've established some good habits.

Starting small is not a cop out it just means that we can genuinely get started. We're not waiting till Monday! We're not waiting till we've eaten all the sweet stuff in the cupboard. We're not waiting until Babs down the road has had her birthday…We're just starting! Do you resonate with the waiting? How many times have you said 'oh I just need to get the dog's birthday out of the way and then I'll start…' If we're always waiting, we will never get there. Life is a series of ups and downs and busyness and that will always be the case so if you're waiting for things

Why W.E.I.G.H.T?

to even out you'll probably be waiting a long time. We have to make things work whatever life is throwing at us!

Check out my 'What's' to get you started!

Takeaways

1. What's your starting point? Do you know where you're starting from? Often, we're so eager to get started we don't take the time to figure out what we're currently doing. Take the time to do this – it will be worth it!
2. What are your non-negotiables? You will have to compromise, but you don't have to sacrifice.
3. What are your goals and are they realistic? If not, you won't stick to them. Reassess before going ahead!
4. What one thing will you start doing today that will make a difference to your progress?

One thing I will start to do from today is…

Chapter Six - Get moving.

I can already hear the groans as you think, 'Oh no, she's going to talk about exercise. I hate exercise. Why do we have to exercise? Well, in order to lose weight, you don't really need to exercise. You can lose weight just by changing your diet. Before you get too excited, if you do add in some exercise to your weight loss plan, you will definitely see the benefits of doing so. Not only that, taking weight loss out of the equation for a second, there are so many benefits to exercise, increased strength, stronger heart, stronger muscles, increased bone density, more confidence, better health… the list goes on!

All these things are going to serve us well in life. I mean, we all want to be able to open our own wine bottles! We're going to need some strength for that. But, seriously we use strength in so many ways during the day; getting in and out of a chair; reaching out to get something from a cupboard; bending down to pick up shopping; picking up children; whatever it may be, and if we do not keep that strength up, we're going to lose it and then as we age, we will find that things become more difficult, even to the point that we may end up needing help with getting around.

So, if you take weight loss out of the equation, movement becomes really important just on its own.

How can it help your weight loss plan?

My S to success framework can help!

Stop being sedentary! Moving more can help increase the number of calories that you're burning. It's all very well doing an exercise class once a week but that's not going to make major changes. It is our day-to-day movement that becomes more important. I mentioned earlier about how much time you might spend sitting down in a day; most of us don't realise how little we're getting up and moving in a day. There are simple ways to increase your daily movement, getting up to make a cup of tea; walking around while the kettle boils; going up the stairs more regularly; not driving everywhere if we don't need to; making sure we're not sat down for long periods of time. All of these things have a massive impact on the number of calories we can burn and if we're doing this sort of thing every day, it's going to have an even bigger impact than just trooping out to one exercise class per week and ticking a box to say done.

If you don't like exercise or you're not ready to exercise yet, adding in this extra movement to your daily life will make a huge difference to your health and to your weight loss.

'I might be thinking about exercise, what would you suggest I try?'

Steps! A really simple way to start your movement off is to just start doing more walking. Walking is an easy and simple thing to do. No equipment is needed, and no special clothing is needed and you can do it whenever the mood grabs you, within reason.

The rest of the people at work might have a bit of an issue if you start banging out squats and bicep curls in the middle of the office, but you'll probably have less of an issue if you just take yourself off for a lunchtime walk!

The good news is you don't have to sprint off like an Olympic speed walker; you can just go for a leisurely walk. You can add a bit more speed if you want to. You can take in some hills if you feel like it. But most of all it is important that you're just getting out there and starting to get those steps in.

You can set yourself mini goals, such as achieving a certain distance, a set time you will walk for or decide a number of steps.

Another thing I try to encourage the women I work with to do is to start strength training.

Strength training (also known as weight training) is about adding extra weight when you're exercising, whether that is using your own body weight, for example push- ups or squats etc or by using things such as dumbbells or kettlebells, or resistance bands. Although this is a book on weight loss and most of us speak about wanting to lose weight what we're really wanting to do is lose fat as this is what will make the biggest difference to our body. Weight loss is just a more general term for this and one that we all understand. You may not believe me, but women will lose fat through strength training despite the scales not moving. The difference is that their body will look completely different from just following a weight loss alone. Generally, that's what most of us want, to look in the mirror and see that change.

I know of many women who've hit their weight loss targets but still aren't happy because it's not quite the desired result they were hoping for, but once they've started adding in that strength training element and seen the difference it can make, they've been much happier with their results.

Strength training will also help with preserving muscle. I can feel your heart rate shooting up already at the thought of walking around like a competitive bodybuilder! When we first start a weight loss plan, we often lose muscle mass. Muscle mass is vital to a successful weight loss or fat loss plan as the more muscle we have, the more calories we're burning at rest.

And don't be scared by the word muscle. You're not going to end up like that bodybuilder! It takes a lot of dedication, a very strict diet and a very specific training plan in order to achieve that kind of physique. If you start lifting weights, I guarantee that you will not get bulky as is the rumour that often goes hand in hand when it comes to women and weight training.

Strength training will also help you to burn fat.

Try not to get sucked into the idea that cardio is the only way forward (cardio is often referring to exercise such as running). You might see a lot of cardio bunnies featured when talking about women's exercise, pictures of women on the treadmill or the cross trainer. When you go to the gym, you'll see that the cross trainers, treadmills and the Stairmasters are largely inhabited by women puffing and sweating their way through a pretty mindless and boring exercise. Okay, that's just my opinion; I admit I'm not the biggest cardio lover.

Why W.E.I.G.H.T?

Of course, if you love that sort of thing, if you love running or cycling, then of course keep it in your plan. It's important that what you're doing is enjoyable, because if you don't enjoy it, you're not going to stick to it, but be open to trying other things as well. Be open to strength training. If you don't do any exercise at the moment, think about what you might be willing to try - maybe you'd enjoy a dance class If you try something and you don't like it, move on to the next thing and give that a try. It's all about finding that thing that's going to get you moving and don't dismiss exercise altogether if the first thing you try doesn't float your boat!

If you're interested in getting into strength training to see what change you can see, then it can be worth getting a professional to support you with this especially if you've never done it before. Learning good technique and form is really important and will serve you well in the future.

Start! So how do you get started? Once again it comes back to picking that one thing you think you can start today.

A 10-minute walk around the block might be the perfect thing to get you started.

Maybe your first step is just visiting the gym to see what it's all about. Seeing what personal trainers are available to help you set up your strength plan doesn't mean that you have to sign up, it just means you're taking those steps to find out.

Taking some sort of action is better than taking no action at all and when we take that first step; it makes us feel good about ourselves and spurs us on to take the next step.

Takeaways

1. Stop being sedentary – movement is key! Daily movement is better than one 45 minute exercise class a week – how can you move more in your day?
2. Steps – walking is the easiest way to get started with movement and open to most of us.
3. Strength – adding in some strength training can really make a change to your body. Get professional help to get started to get the best results.
4. Start – what will you start doing today to increase your movement?

I will increase my movement by...

Chapter 7 - Habits

How many times have you heard knowledge is power? Of course having knowledge is powerful, but do you know what is more powerful? Action!

Habits are simply actions that you take regularly to move you towards your goals.

Some habits we do because we know we should, for example, cleaning our teeth. Some habits we do because we're getting an incentive, for example, getting up and going to work because we get paid and we have bills! Who came up with this whole adulting thing anyway?

Some habits are better for us, for example, drinking water and some habits not so good for us such as smoking.

For some reason, we often find it hard to instil good habits into our daily routine especially if they're new habits. Let's say we decide we're going to start exercising or eating more fruit and veg, it can seem like a really hard thing to do, but if I told you to eat more cake or sit down on the sofa more, you'd probably find that a much easier task!

Usually, we associate good habits with things that we consider to be a chore, or we might not enjoy as much. I mean, who wouldn't love to be told they needed to eat more cake?

Those less healthy habits generally seem to require a lot less effort than those healthier habits that we're actually trying to make a part of our life. It can also feel that good habits take a lot longer to establish. However, bad habits that we've acquired also have usually taken us quite a while to do; we just weren't paying as much attention because they felt nicer!

If we think about gaining weight, it isn't something that happened overnight, it was a result of lots of things done over a period of time that lead us to gain weight.

If we think how we became more sedentary, we didn't just decide one day to sit down more often and that we weren't going to be as active anymore. It was, again, a series of things that happened over a period of time that led us to become more sedentary.

The exact same thing happens when we try to increase our healthier habits.

It's foolish to expect that we can go from not drinking any water or not eating any fruit and veg or not doing any exercise to suddenly be hitting all our proposed targets after day one or even week one. They're going to take time to build just like our bad habits that we built over a period of time. When we're trying to build good habits, we often have a goal in mind, or we know that our good habits are leading us to something that we want, such as weight loss. Bad habits generally don't have the same goal-oriented outcome.

Now you might think you'll be more incentivised if you've got a goal to aim for. It's logical right? The trouble is that our goals often seem out of reach, as we've already covered in this book, so the end goal seems like it's so far away that we start the good habits, but when we're still not hitting the goal, we become deflated and give up. Instead of thinking of the habits in their own right we're only thinking them of them in relation to the goal. This means if we don't achieve the goal, we give up on the habit.

We need to take the goal or the outcome away from the habits that we're trying to build. Someone once said to me that in order to achieve good things, we need to detach from the outcome. They used a specific acronym, NATO, which has stuck with me and stands for Not Attached To Outcome. This basically refers to the fact that we don't actually have any control over the outcome. So you could do all the right things to become a millionaire and still not become a millionaire. But along the way, you most definitely would have made some gains. You might not be a millionaire, but you're probably going to have more money than you would have done had you not put into place the habits needed to become a millionaire.

If you were so focused on the outcome of becoming a millionaire, but every time you didn't become one you gave up you'd probably be no better off than when you started. And this is the same when we're applying habits to weight loss. It can be really hard to detach from the outcome, the weight loss goal, but if we can detach from it, we allow ourselves to put our focus back on the habits and the daily actions that we need to do which are the important bit. Without habits and actions you don't have a plan to build on.

If you're doing this, if you're completing your daily actions, those regular habits, you'll probably find that you will get the results that you want anyway.

Let's look at another example.

Athletes train, day in day out, they follow a specific diet and they follow all the things they need to do to win at their sport. However, doing all the things that they need to do to win at their sport doesn't necessarily mean that they are going to win at their sport. But it doesn't stop them continuing to do those daily tasks, following their nutrition and exercise plan because they know by doing that, they're more likely to win at their sport than if they weren't doing those tasks.

Now, if we can put this in relation to your weight loss - say your desired outcome was to lose two stone, you could start putting some habits into place such as eating more fruit and veg, upping your protein, increasing the amount of daily movement you did, drinking more water and looking at your sleep patterns. Then you could weigh yourself a couple of weeks later and find out that you hadn't lost any weight and you could give up deciding those habits weren't working and go back to your old ways. Or you could continue with those habits despite the fact that you didn't really see any change on the scale, forget about the two stone outcome and what you will probably find in the end is that you would either lose the two stone or be much closer to it than if you had given up altogether. You will have enjoyed the journey a lot more because you wouldn't have been obsessing over the end result.

Let's talk about habits in more detail. What do you need to be doing? What does that look like?

Habits should always be things that you **can** achieve and if you can fit them into your day to make it easier for you to remember to do them, then so much the better. For example, what can you do at the same time as other things you do every day, such as cleaning your teeth? Can you put another action in place at that time, one that will move you towards your goal? You could drink a glass of water before you clean your teeth or eat a piece of fruit whilst the kettle boils. Why put a new habit with an old one? Because if it's something you're regularly doing it means you won't have to think too much about doing the new habit. You know you're going to clean your teeth in the morning before you go to work so have a glass of water ready to drink first – great one glass of water ticked off the list and you barely had to give it a thought!

We also want habits to be realistic. If like me, you're not a morning person setting a new habit for a 10-minute walk at 6am is probably unlikely and even if you do it for the first few days; you may not carry on with it. I once went for a 6am walk – just once!!!

If you feel more alive at midday or 4pm or 6pm then scheduling in a 10 minute walk at that time would be much more realistic and achievable for you as an individual.

It doesn't matter that your smug friend gets up at 5am does a 30 minute workout, prepares a stew to put in the slow cooker and does two loads of washing before they go to work. If you're not a morning person it's not going to be successful for you without making a lot of effort (take it from someone who knows). The way to succeed at losing weight and to keep it off is to make it as simple for yourself at that time. If you do want to become the sort of person that gets up at 5am we can worry about that later down the line. Let's focus on what you can do now and then we can move on from there. (P.S. don't tell your friend I told her she was smug, I'm just jealous that she's more organised than me).

It's also important not to worry if you miss a day with your habit. Remember, it's all a work in progress to start with, you're not expected to be perfect. Focus on progress and building those habits bit by bit.

Maybe day one you got up and drank water when you cleaned your teeth. Day two you didn't. That doesn't mean you stop because it didn't work out. It means that day three, you just do it again. Day four you do it again. If you miss day five, you do it on day six and so often, by continuing with the habits, eventually you will do it without even thinking about it and you'll become more and more consistent as time goes on.

Thinking specifically about your weight loss what habits do you need to be putting in place?

Here are some of my suggestions for good habits to get started with.

1. Think about drinking more water. What can you successfully manage – maybe one glass a day or just increasing what you are already drinking?
2. Eat more protein. Protein can be things like meat, fish, eggs, vegan and vegetarian alternatives such as Quorn. Protein helps you to feel fuller for longer and is also one of the building blocks of the body helping with muscle repair and growth.
3. Eat more fruit and vegetables. Ideally, you want half of your dinner plate to be vegetables. This is easier to do than you might think. 80 grams of vegetables is one portion and you'll be surprised at how small this portion is. So, it's a lot easier to hit your five a day than you think. An easy way to hit your 5 a day do this is to have a portion of fruit and veg with your breakfast, two at lunch and two at dinner. Remember, five is not the maximum number it's the minimum so if you want to pile in more veg to your day, then go ahead.
4. Add more movement. We've already spoken about this in the previous chapter, but it can be really easy to fall into bad habits of spending lots of time sitting down. Again, movement doesn't have to be scary. It can be as simple as going out for a walk, being

more active at home, getting up from your desk more often etc. Think about how you can start to implement movement into your day and make this a habit.

5. Get enough sleep! Now, you may be thinking how does sleep fit into my weight loss plan? I've never had this suggested at any of the slimming clubs I've been to. Sleep is important for many reasons. If we don't get enough sleep, we'll often find that our stress levels are elevated. We may also feel hungrier as lack of sleep leads to the release of a hormone called ghrelin – the hunger hormone. This can lead to us making poor food choices because we're too tired to think about cooking a meal or working out what to eat. If we're well rested, we're more likely to make better choices. If we're tired, we may be less inclined to do more movement which can also affect our weight loss.

There are many habits that you can start to implement that will support your weight loss goals but the key to successfully get habits underway is to not take on too many at one time. Pick one and work on it until you're happy with it, until it becomes part of your life and then move on to another one.

Trying to implement everything at once will only lead to you feeling overwhelmed and potentially giving up which is what we want to avoid. We've been there, we've done that. This time we're doing it for life!

Takeaways

1. Start small! It's better to take one habit and do it well than do 10 half-heartedly.
2. Pick something that's easy for you to do to start with – if you pledge to do cold water swimming every morning, but you hate water and the cold, probably not going to work! Say you will drink a glass of water while the kettle boils – much more doable!
3. Look at your sleep habits – are you getting enough and what can you do to improve it?

The first habit I will start to implement is…

Chapter 8 – The 4 Ts

And finally, the last part of my framework the 4 Ts.

The first T is **trust**. You have to learn to trust yourself again! Dieting mentality has made you feel that you can't trust yourself around certain foods. You can't trust yourself to know when you're full up. You can't trust yourself to know when you're hungry. You can't trust yourself to go down the sweet aisle at Sainsbury's, (other supermarkets are available). It's craziness! You can trust yourself and you have to learn to trust your decisions once again.

You also have to trust that you want to do the best for yourself. If you feel that you want to do the best for yourself you're more likely to make decisions that support that, for example you're more likely to eat well most of the time and remember, that's all we're aiming for – most of the time! None of us are perfect and if we were eating perfectly all the time, it would be a rigid life. I know people who eat the same thing day in day out. They won't ever have a biscuit or chocolate or a cake because they're so brainwashed by some of the slimming clubs that they've attended. I just look at this and think imagine never being able

to have a chocolate covered Hobnob again or have a spoon of Nutella out of the jar. It's not for me that's for sure!

If you learn to trust yourself again, you'll know that you can have those things, but you'll also know that you are not going to eat the whole packet of chocolate covered hobnobs or scrape the Nutella jar dry. If those things do happen sometimes, say you do scoff the whole packet of chocolate covered hobnobs, then you'll trust that actually tomorrow you won't need to do it again, you will go back to whatever you were doing before and it will be just fine.

You also need to trust the process which brings me on to my next T which is about **time**. Most of us are looking to do things in the quickest time possible in the easiest way possible but that's just not real life. We can make things as simple as we can, of course, but generally, it's hard to do good things quickly. We need to take our time with them and the whole point of losing weight and keeping it off is to embed habits, actions and mindset into our lives that will remain with us for a long time and that's going to take practice and practice needs time in order to work. If we think about the fact that time is going to pass anyway, whether we do or don't do the things we need to, we might as well be doing them and we might as well take our time. All those diets that you started for a few weeks and managed to get some results, chances are that after another few weeks, you were back at the beginning and starting the process again. This is precisely what we're trying to avoid this time around. We're trying to avoid yo-yoing and going back to square one. It can be hard to trust a process that seems longer than we're used to or longer than we've been told we should be used to. And this is where trust is really going to come into play.

If you give something enough time, with the skills that you're learning through this book, you will find that the results will outweigh the amount of time that you've spent on them. And let's remember, it didn't take you a few weeks or a few days to put the weight on.

This has happened over a long period of time so we need to allow the same time in order to lose the weight as well.

As I've mentioned several times in this book, if we're trying to rush something, the chances are that we're doing it in a very restrictive and miserable way. We're trying to avoid that way of weight loss because we want it to be sustainable. We want to be able to maintain what we're doing for the rest of our lives so that we're not constantly caught in this dieting trap we've probably found ourselves in for goodness knows how many years.

Another factor with time is to stop waiting. The time will never be right for you to start your weight loss plan. There will always be something as we've mentioned, it might be the cat getting their degree, or your kid's birthdays, or a relative's wedding, or your friend turns 50… Whatever it might be, something is always going to come up, so the time is never going to be perfect, but time is very rarely perfect in life for anything. Stop saying you're going to start when whatever thing is over and just say that you're going to start today. It doesn't matter what you start with. You could start by drinking that extra glass of water. You could start by going for that five-minute walk. You could start by having an extra piece of veg with your dinner. All of those things are perfectly doable while life goes on.

My third T tip is all about **treats** - the good stuff. Now I'm not that keen on the word treat when it comes to weight loss because I think it automatically sets up that thinking in your mind that it is something you shouldn't have. However, we don't want weight loss to be boring. We don't want weight loss to be miserable. So, it's important that we make sure that we have some sort of treat every day. Now a treat does not have to be something that we eat. It could be doing something nice for us. It could also, of course, be something that we eat. As I mentioned earlier in the book, one of my non-negotiables is that I can have my two chocolate biscuits a day. Sometimes I have them, sometimes I don't. It's absolutely fine to make a certain food part of your plan if you enjoy it just keep it all in moderation and balance. The whole Victoria sponge or a three foot long tiger loaf would count as more than a treat but you get where I'm going with this.

So maybe you will decide that chocolate bar you always have at lunchtime is a non-negotiable for you and that is your daily treat, it's something you're going to look forward to and it is going to allow you to stay on track with your weight loss plan. Or it might be that you decide that your treat is going to be something purely for you. Losing weight is about doing something to make you feel good to improve your health. Maybe your treat is to have the bath with the candles and the rose petals and read your book while no one disturbs you. It might be that your treat is to settle down with a cup of tea in your pyjamas and watch an episode of the boxset that you've been putting off for the last five years. Whatever your treat is, make sure you include something every day, it doesn't have to be the same thing, mix it up! All the time you know you've got nice things in your life, you're more likely to be committed to taking those steps to a successful weight loss plan.

Treat tip: Write a selection of treats on bits of paper and put them in a jar and pick one out each day to give you the surprise factor!

My final T is to **turn up** for yourself. At the end of the day, the only one who is going to do this is you. No one else is going to be able to lose weight for you, to do the actions that need to be done in order to lose weight or to make the food choices that need to be made in order to lose weight - only you.

Once you accept this, you're taking ownership of the choices you're making which is so important. Often many of us are used to making excuses for why things aren't happening. I know I've been guilty of it myself. Saying I haven't got time, I'm too busy for whatever it is that I'm making an excuse for, but it's not that at all, I'm just not prioritising that thing. Maybe whatever you need to do feels too big so you feel you can't do it or maybe you're not sure where to start. If you want to succeed, you need to stop saying those things and acknowledge that the only one who's going to make this happen is you. This is your new thought process, it's not about 'If you want it badly enough, you'll do it' type speech because sometimes we do want things badly, but our mindset isn't in the right place to achieve it. This is about saying that if you want it you are going to turn up for yourself every day in some way however that looks. It could be small steps like the ones we've spoken about earlier in the book or it may be in bigger ways like joining a gym or signing up to an online fitness membership. You are worth turning up for you and by doing the things that you need to do, you're going to be reinforcing that mantra within yourself, which is going to be great for your confidence, great for your self-esteem and great for your self-worth.

Takeaways

1. Trust! Learn to trust yourself again. You can say no to that extra piece of cake. You might not want to, but you can!
2. Time! The process will take time if it's going to work. It can be hard if you don't see immediate results like the ones you might get with many slimming club programmes. The process is about long-term success, not short-term gains and that's what we want!
3. Treats! Treat yourself! Knowing you can have what you like in your weight loss plan is one of the keys to the success of that plan. Don't restrict everything – compromise!
4. Turn up! Do something every day that shows you that you matter and is taking you a step closer to the person you want to be.

FAQs

What if I don't have the money to buy fancy ingredients for weight loss meals?

That's exactly one of the reasons why I wanted to write this book, to show you that you don't have to do anything fancy. I will not be telling you to buy chia seeds or only drink the milk of a rare yeti found only in the Himalayas. Remember, we are trying to lose weight for life so we need the food we eat to be choices we can stick to and that's going to look different for everyone. Maybe you love the milk of a rare yeti or maybe you're happy with more traditional dinners! When we individualise your plan you can take your budget into account.

Do I have to give up cakes, biscuits and sweets?

No! What are you thinking?? Now, of course there will need to be some sort of compromise – you can't eat lots of 'treat' foods on top of your normal diet and expect to see the weight loss results you want, but it's unrealistic to expect that you are never going to eat those things again, so we make them a part of your plan! Simples! No need to go without to get the results you want.

How will I know what portions to eat?

Portions can be a tricky thing – we're so used to seeing big helpings of everything these days, super sizing and adding extras it can be hard to know what our plates should look like. However, if you are currently overeating, we want to make sure you reduce your portion sizes appropriately so you don't feel extreme hunger which can lead to binges. This is where it's helpful to look at your starting point and figuring out what you're currently eating and that's exactly what we do when we individualise your plan! You will also be able to use my success plate to help you gauge the correct portions.

How do you successfully lose weight when you're busy?

It's something I hear a lot 'I'm so busy/too busy'. Hell, I even say it myself… a lot!!! Life is busy these days – I hear ya! But life will always be busy in one way or another and it's finding a plan that works with the way your lifestyle looks. Maybe you don't have time to cook freshly made meals each day – that's ok; you can factor that in and still make choices that support your goals. This is where really figuring out what works for you is key – if I tell you to cook home-made meals with a 13-page recipe each day you're more than likely going to fall at the first hurdle, but finding a sensible option that you know you can stick to most of the time is the one for the win!

What do I do if I don't have time to workout?

Get down and give me 20! Just kidding, but that's probably a little bit of what you think when you hear 'workout'. Remember that we are reframing exercise! It really is about movement and more of it in your daily life! Everyone has time to move more in the day – unless someone has stapled you to your chair! You don't need to schedule in exercise time just make sure you're sitting down less. Again, think about what works for you, because that is the secret to success.

How do I stay on track with my eating when I'm busy?

By making a plan that works for you. One size does not fit all and remember you don't need any special foods or ways of eating to achieve your weight loss goals. Also, cut yourself some slack! There will be times when maybe it doesn't all go to plan, but if you've got a good system in place to follow you will find it much easier. My W.E.I.G.H.T system has all the tools you need to stay on track.

How do I overcome my mindset, so I stop giving up?

The mindset is the most important part so it's a great question. It's also the part we probably need to do the most work on and that's why we really focus on that as part of my W.E.I.G.H.T system. Ridding ourselves of some of those diet myths and limiting beliefs and changing how we think about weight loss will help you see better results in no time.

You make it sound so easy; can I really make better choices?

Yes, you can! It really is just a case of starting small and working up from there. Remember this is a marathon not a sprint and we don't need to work on everything all at once! Also, you will be more likely to make better choices if you know you're not giving everything up!

I am an emotional eater; will this stop me succeeding?

No, it just means we need to do a bit of work on the mindset elements. 99% of the time we don't feel any better when we emotionally eat, but by looking at our reasons why, setting new habits and putting them into action you can overcome this.

I would love to have more 1-2-1 help with my weight loss, but I don't think I can afford it.

Sometimes we all need some extra help! And sometimes that does come at an extra cost, but you need to weigh up the benefits. What will it do for you? Will it make it more likely that you will succeed? What will success look like? Having someone in your corner guiding you in the right direction could be just what you need.

What makes your book different?

Because we create your individual weight loss plan, not a plan that is churned out to everyone. Because we are looking at your individual circumstances you will come away with a weight loss plan that perfectly suits your lifestyle and that you can sustain!

Isn't that complicated though?

No! In fact, it couldn't be simpler because it works with the diet you have and the lifestyle you lead. We always start from there and make changes that fit. Done for you meal plans just don't work for long term weight loss but putting you in charge of the changes does!

What are the obstacles you might face along the way?

Now there is one thing that could prevent your success with your weight loss plan after reading this book, and that is if you find yourself slipping back into that old diet mindset. We've already established that it hasn't helped you in the past and it's not going to help you moving forward. I totally understand how easy it is to slip back into something that you know, something that you feel has worked because you have lost weight on it. However, you didn't manage to lose the weight and keep it off. That diet mindset can easily draw us back into looking at the quick fixes and the generic done for you plans - it's comfortable there. We know it. Trying something new is always daunting but what we need to remind ourselves is that if we really want to achieve success with our weight loss, it's going to take more time than we've probably spent previously on individual diets, diet clubs, diet plans, whichever route you followed in the past, but think about how much time you've spent collectively but still not getting the results, is it really going to be so bad to spend time on something different?

As we've already spoken about, we're constantly presented with adverts for the next weight loss plan, the next big fad and it can be hard to stay focused on what we're doing when something around the corner seems shinier and newer. In order to overcome these setbacks, what do you need to do? You need to believe in the process, put your trust in something new and see if it works for you. Don't decide after one or two weeks that nothing's happening and so you're going to give up. Getting where you want to be takes time. You didn't put on the weight in a couple of weeks and you're not realistically going to lose it in a couple of weeks. The reason we lose a lot of weight when we first attend a slimming club is because we lose water and muscle. What we want to be doing is losing fat and that's exactly what this book and my W.E.I.G.H.T framework will help you to do. That is what will get you the best results. You will see those results when you look in the mirror and you will feel better for it.

Secondly, you need to be consistent if you're going to follow something new and trust the process. And this is not the same as being perfect. It's about being consistent most of the time. There are always going to be days when things don't go to plan, or we don't follow what we've set out to, but it's about not letting that push you back and start that failure type thinking, 'well I've blown it now, I might as well give up'. The other way to overcome it is to find a group of people who are there to support you, to support your accountability, to help you when those times get hard and you feel like moving on to that shiny new diet that you saw a reality show celebrity gushing over on Instagram. Having people around you who understand what you're trying to achieve and are fully supportive will really help keep you on the path that you're trying to follow. This has really succeeded for some of the women I've worked with; by joining my groups they found women that can empathise with them and help them when they hit those low times.

They've also developed the mindset to know that it's ok to not be perfect all the time and accepting that and moving on is really one of the major success points to losing weight and keeping it off because they no longer have to start from the beginning every time they hit a little bump in the road.

So, how do you get started?

I appreciate that you want to just get on with things and see results as quickly as possible. I want that for you too! But more than that I want you to get results and maintain them and that's why it's important you do the steps in the book.

I really want you to start working on your mindset, beginning with working through those diet myths you may have ingested. Take your time to think about whether they have served you in the past.

However, there are some things you can start doing immediately to start accelerating your results.

1. Add more fruit and vegetables into your diet.
2. Increase your water intake.
3. Start moving more – think about your steps!
4. Watch your portion sizes!

Let's recap on what you need to work through for the best results: -

W – Weed out the BS! Work through those diet myths and see how much of this information you've absorbed and what hasn't worked for you. Determine what your own limiting beliefs are – how are they holding you back?

E – Enjoy food again! Stop calling foods 'good' and 'bad' and just think about how you can make changes to your current diet that means you're not over restricting but you are making changes that serve you in your current lifestyle. Make sure that you are deciding which foods you don't want to give up – your non-negotiables and probably most importantly, keep the changes simple so that you can sustain them.

Why W.E.I.G.H.T?

I – Individualise your plan! This is the part where you start thinking about what is really going to work for you and your lifestyle and building your plan. Firstly, you need to know where you're starting – this is so important. If you don't know this information, how will you know what to do next? Make sure you set realistic goals, remember we want to keep this weight off and realistic and achievable goals will help you to do this. Remember we are compromising, not sacrificing!

G – Get moving! I know, exercise urgh!! Remember there's more ways to move than squats and push ups (although these movements are important, but that's a different book)! Just being less sedentary in your everyday life is the key to keeping active and burning those calories. It really is as simple as starting to increase your steps.

H – Habits! Like with everything, simple really is better. Think about habits you can thread into your normal life and stick to. If necessary, just pick one habit and do it well before moving on to the next one. Don't forget your sleep habits too. Sleep, or lack of, can have a huge effect on our weight loss.

T – The 4 Ts! Trust, Time, Treats, Turn up for yourself. This might be hard, but you need to trust the process if you want to see results. It can be so easy to fall back into old habits, but you're here for a reason, reading this book and still trying to figure out the secrets to your weight loss. Within that, you need to trust that it's going to take time. Losing weight and keeping it off is not a quick process, in fact the quicker it is the less likely you are to be able to keep the weight off. Don't forget to treat yourself – it's important that you include foods and activities you enjoy during your weight loss plan. Turning up – you are the only one who can do this. You can get support and accountability, but ultimately it's down to you so let's make this the year you start turning up for you!

I would love to hear how you get on so please keep me posted on your success at fitwithleanne@gmail.com.

What now?

Need a bit more help or want to continue your journey? There are more ways to work with me…

Fancy a 1-2-1 chat with me to get you started? Book a 30 minute consultation here www.bookwhen.com/thefemalefitclub

Join my free Facebook group for more tips and advice-
https://www.facebook.com/groups/thefemalefitclub/.

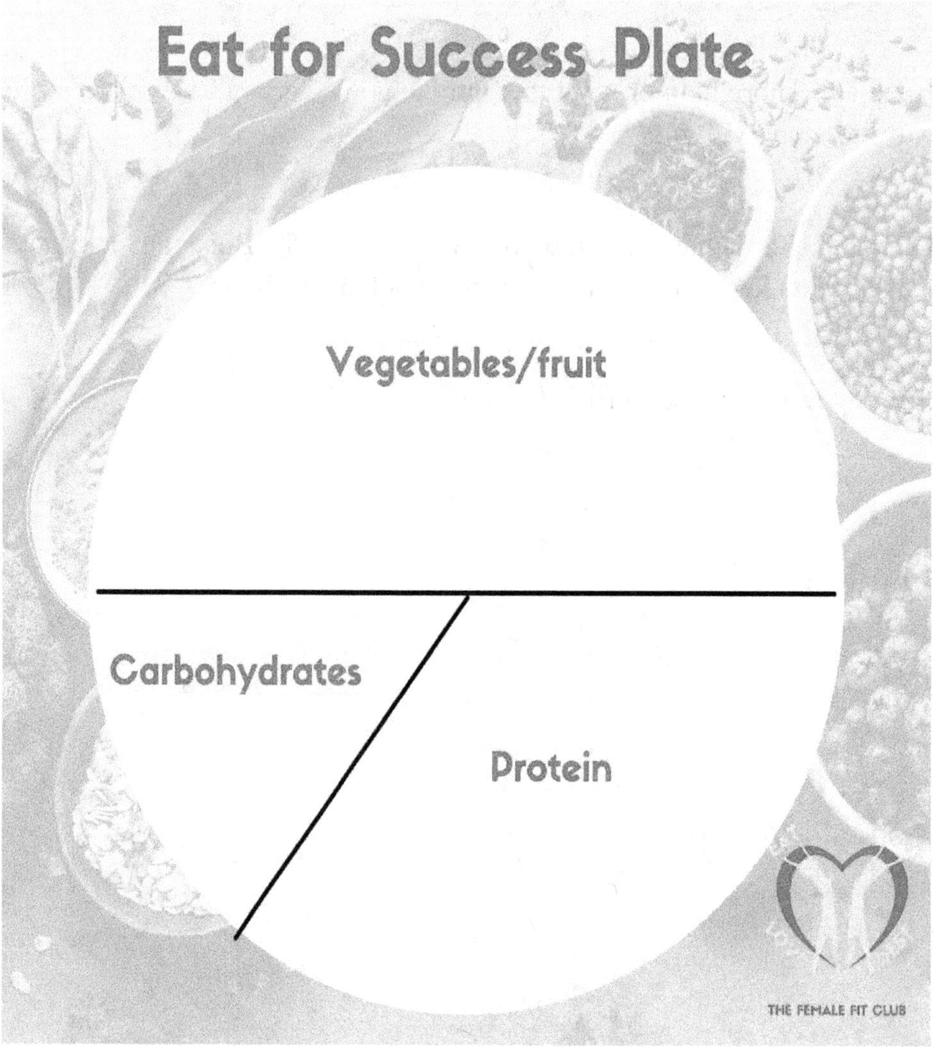

Eat for Success Plate

About the Author

Leanne has been in the fitness industry for over 20 years, winning several awards along the way. She has trained as both an Exercise to Music instructor and Personal Trainer, as well as undertaking specialist education on the menopause.

She is the creator of The Female Fit Club, designed to support women with their weight loss, health and fitness goals both online and in person.

Leanne has written numerous articles for magazines and been a contributing writer to two other books.

Away from work Leanne enjoys the odd prosecco, reading, going to concerts and buying pink things! The first thing Leanne does when getting home is put on her much loved slippers. She has one daughter and a pampered cat!